Herbal Medicines on the Santa Fe Trail

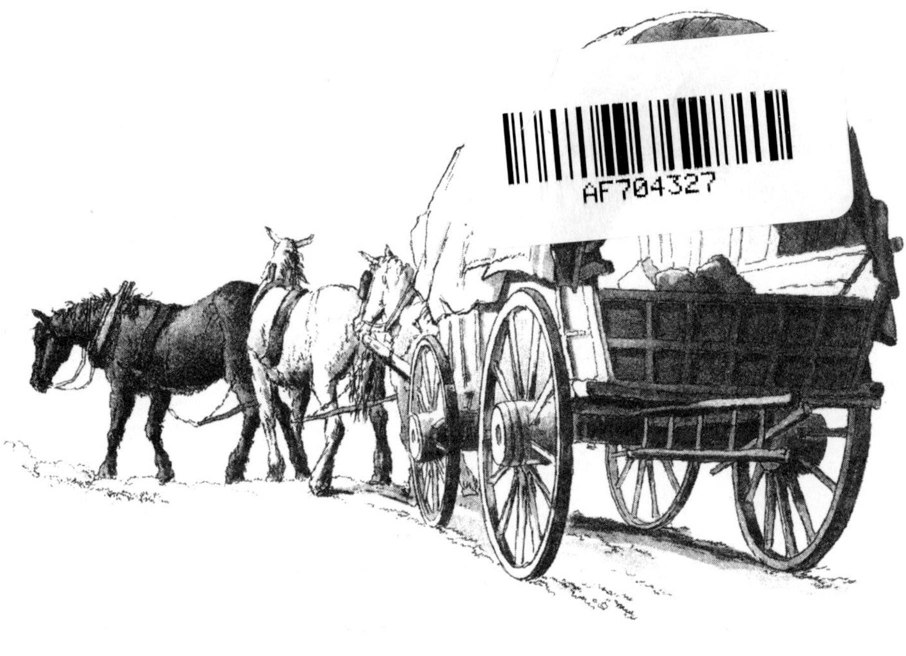

Jim Long

Long Creek Herbs
P.O. Box 127
Blue Eye, Missouri 65611
www.Longcreekherbs.com

Herbal Medicines on the Santa Fe Trail

A Brief Look at the Plants & Medicines in Use
Between 1820 and 1860

Long Creek Herbs
P.O. Box 127
Blue Eye, Missouri 65611
www.Longcreekherbs.com

Printed in the United States by Paul's Printing

ISBN #1-889791-08-3

Expanding Commerce Westward

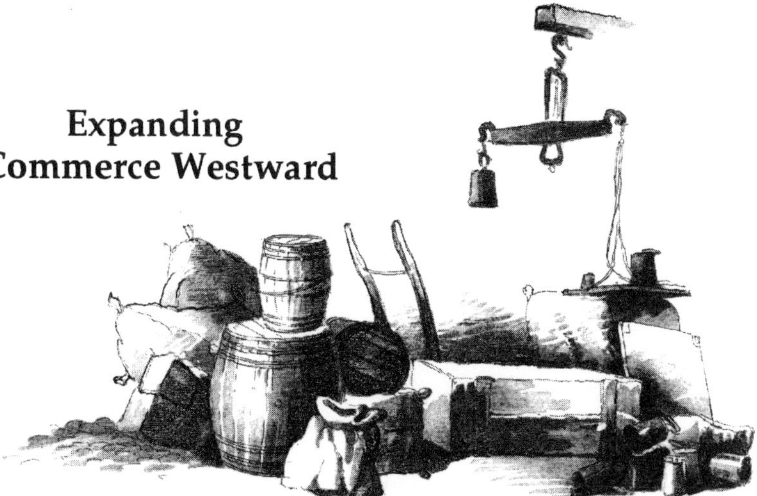

The Santa Fe Trail was primarily about commerce. Wagon trains loaded with materials to sell headed west, into Indian Territory. Traders took cloth and gunpowder from St. Louis and traded those for buffalo hides to take back east on return trips, selling them in St. Louis. An expanding population sought new land, traders wanted new markets and adventurers looked for gold, silver and easy prosperity.

Wines from France and vermillion and tea from China were transported by wagon train in casks and barrels and boxes. Hard bread, baked in St. Louis, was carried in crates to be sold in supply stores. Glass beads in several colors, from Italy, went on the Trail and were traded to native people for animal pelts. Soap, whiskey and cones, or "hats," of sugar, were carried. Brass buttons, more expensive and fashionable than the hand-made coin buttons, were carried to the forts and supply stores, along with muslin, silk and wool. Blankets, shoes, boots, guns, canteens, nails, ink and medicines, all were carried on the wagon trains to supply the migrations of people heading into the "new" land.

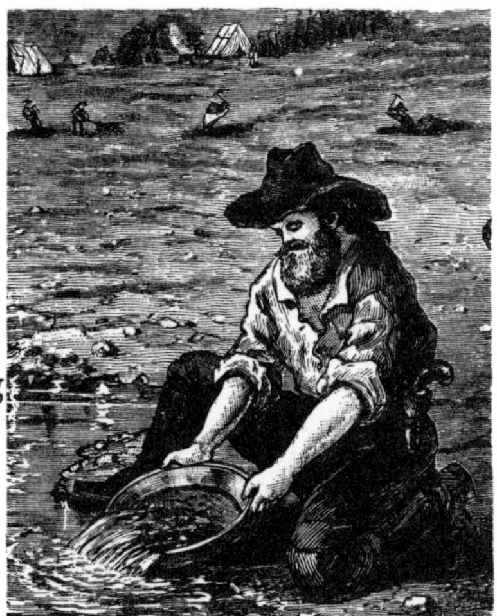

Some went to trade, some to regain their health and some went to chase prosperity.

People struck out on the Trail for varying purposes. Some went to make their fortunes as traders, setting up supply stores along the trail, or even building private forts, like the privately-owned Ft. Bent. Some went for freedom from the congestion of a growing population in the central portion of the country, while others traveling the Trail went to look for gold or silver. Some left home because of illness, seeking a more agreeable climate in which to heal.

It was this migration of people who suffered from tuberculosis, measles, cholera and malaria, that quickly spread disease on the Trail.

Soldiers, sent to protect new settlements, brought with them the diseases caused by unsanitary conditions from living in close quarters without good food and water. Disease spread by way of the trade routes, down the rivers and along the trails from settlement to settlement.

With no knowledge about germs, bacteria or sterilization, illness could move rapidly within groups of settlers. People mistakenly believed that "miasma," invisible vapors from swamps and low places, were the real causes of disease. Eating unsalted beef, bathing too often, exposure to the weather and disruption of the humors, were all held accountable for illness.

Water

> "The road is very badly supplied with water. From our last night's camp we came only five or six miles before stopping...learning from other traders encamped here that we should find no more for some twelve miles."
>
> From the *Diary of Susan Shelby Magoffin*, 1847

Water was obtained wherever it could be found along the Trail. Streams, creeks, rivers or potholes were all utilized for drinking purposes. Horses and men drank from the same streams. In areas where malaria had not been known previously, one infected person might start an outbreak, infecting the mosquitoes which bit them, and the mosquitoes, in turn, infecting more people.

Most of the westward expansion of the United States took place on, or near, rivers. The rivers served as the main transportation and trade routes for both goods and people and the slow speeds of the river journeys allowed for infections and disease to spread rapidly. When travelers for the west left the Missouri River at Westport, at the start of the Santa Fe Trail, rivers remained a major component of travel. Trails followed

> "He became sick with chills and fever, a sickness in which I truly sympathize...experience has taught me that the shaking and quaking of bones is not a very agreeable sensation. I must therefore turn his nurse and relieve if possible a brother sufferer - first here is 'Sappington's celebrated fever and ague pills'."
>
> *Susan Magoffin, Sept. 26, 1847*

rivers, crossed them, and people camped near them, relying upon their waters for sustenance. Malaria, prevalent throughout the entire Mississippi Valley, was soon transported along the westward trails by already sick and suffering people. Even though malaria was not known earlier in New Mexico, by 1848 it was common, showing up regularly on military medical reports.

Known as intermittent fever, the ague, bilious fever, miasmal or marsh fever and many other names, malaria was difficult to cure. Daniel Drake, a doctor in Cincinnati, Ohio, wrote in 1830, "...that there is a noxious gas given out throughout the great Mississippi Valley system which affects the people of the west and south." Writing again in 1850 in his book, *Diseases of the Interior Valley of North America,* he ranks malaria as the most important disease in North America and describes its prevalence throughout the Mississippi Valley, from Wheeling, Pennsylvania on the Ohio River, to New Orleans, to Chicago, down to Arrow Rock and Lexington, Missouri. Still another physician, Dr. Farrar of St. Louis, was quoted as saying that he could distinguish the settlers of the lowlands opposite St. Louis by their perpetually pale and always sickly appearance.

Malaria, when not treated, might subside for awhile, leaving the patient weak and pale, with the disease returning, bringing intermittent fever, chills and diarrhea.

The medical thought of the day was that the patient should be given powerful emetics to cause vomiting, along with strong compounds to cause purging. Those, combined with frequent blood-letting, were claimed to be the best remedies. Even though Peruvian bark was available, doctors disagreed about its use. Most, in the 1830s and 1840s, believed that the bark should only be given on days when the patient did not have fever, and only then after severe purging and bleeding.

Even as late as the Civil War, malaria was causing more sickness and death among the troops of both armies than any other single disease. In the history of Saline County, Missouri, 1881, records show that an early settlement in that area was abandoned because of the prevalence of the "shaking agues." The histories of other counties along the Missouri and Mississippi Rivers show similar fates for many early settlements.

Thomas B. Hall, M.D. wrote in 1930, "While we have no exact statistical data available it is probable that in many communities the infection with the disease was at or near one hundred percent of the population. During the months of July, August and September (the sickly season), when malaria was most rife, the conditions were appalling...There was scarcely a family which did not have one or more of its members stricken, and in many instances, the well were hard put to take care of the sick and dying."

All kinds of remedies for the ague abounded. Writing in his diary in 1859, at age 18, Elias Slagle recorded this remedy for the Ague:

"Take a piece of muslin or any thin goods and cut it so it will cover the back from neck to hips, and about the width of the back; then take common cotton batting and tack it on so it will be about an inch in thickness, and put it on to the necked back and wear it there for 2 or 3 months and you will have no more ague. Never know it to fail."

The innocence of this remedy points up both the futility of many of the folk remedies for malaria as well as the ignorance of the progression of the disease. Covering the body with cloth and leaving it there for 2 or 3 months tells us two things: (1) People weren't aware that the disease would run its course and would subside during the winter months (thus the "never fail" remedy for those who lived through the first course of the disease suffered its return with intermittent fever and illness that lasted for several seasons); and, (2) people didn't bathe often. There was the belief that water on the body could cause all kinds of maladies and other remedies in the same diary record the caution to avoid water on the body at every opportunity.

Quinine was used in Peru by native people for centuries, but two Jesuit missionaries are credited with its "discovery" in the late 1700s. Known as "Peruvian bark," it was introduced in Europe, and two French chemists, Pelletier and Caventon isolated quinine from the bark in 1820. Before that time, the use of the bark was not predictable as more than one species of tree offered the medicine-containing bark, and strengths of the medicine varied from batch to batch. Also, as is often the case when money is concerned, traders who transported the bark often adulterated it with other bark, increasing their profits out of greed. By 1830, pure quinine was being manufactured in Philadelphia and it was known that malaria could be quickly controlled if a patient was given quinine.

But because not much was known about malaria, and because medicine of the day was wrought with supersition, tradition and ignorance, the official and accepted treatment seems wasteful and horrendous to us today. Doctors practiced copious bloodletting, purging and vomiting of their malaria patients before beginning treatment with quinine. It was believed at the time that bleeding the patient was more important than the administering of the remedy, and doctors would bleed the patient many times over a 3 or 4 day period, following each with medicines that caused severe evacuation of the bowels, then violent vomiting. Only when the patient was exhausted after nearly a week of this, would the quinine be administered. Many patients already desperately ill with malaria, didn't live long enough to receive the real medicine.

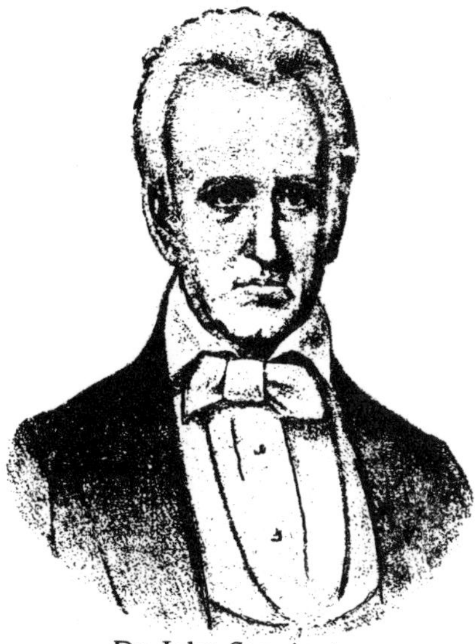
Dr. John Sappington

Dr. Sappington's Anti-Fever Pills

Dr. John Sappington moved to Missouri in 1817, already a practicing physician. He had received his training as an apprentice with his father, who was also a doctor, and had studied medicine at the University of Pennyslvania.

He had been influenced greatly by the early writings of Dr. Henry Perrine, who had written in 1826, just six years after quinine had been isolated from Peruvian bark, that quinine was a specific for malarial fevers and should be administered immediately at the onset of the disease. Further, he did not hold to the practice of bleeding and purging. Sappington had opposed those practices from the beginning of his medical career.

Dr. Sappington practiced medicine in Howard County, Missouri for two years, then moved across the river to Saline County, near Arrow Rock. Because of his success with the treatment of the ague, his reputation spread rapidly. He often traveled 100 miles or more on horseback to see his patients. (It is said that in order to make better use of his time while traveling, he carried bags of bluegrass seed on the back of his saddle, scattering it along the trails as he rode. Some of that early bluegrass that he brought with him from Tennessee and planted, still grows in that part of the state.)

As he was in the area where malaria was common, he had cause to try out Dr. Perrine's recommendations often and found that he could rely on quinine alone to cure malaria. He became a vigorous promoter of quinine as a true and effective remedy for this disease and his endorsement of the drug is seen in his statement, "The names of Pelletier and Caventon, who first separated the pure alkaline salt, called quinine, from the bulky and inert mass in which nature had placed it, deserve to be remembered with grattitude by all mankind."

But the medical schools of the day continued to recommend the barbarous customs of bloodletting and purging, even releasing statements chastising Sappington for his "frivolous treatments," warning physicians to avoid his advice.

In 1832 Dr. Sappington began the manufacturing of anti-fever pills. Each pill contained one grain of quinine, three-fourths of a grain of licorice and one-fourth grain of myrrh, with some oil of sassafras for flavoring. The sale of the pills became so brisk that he had difficulties keeping up with demand and soon expanded his operation.

He began distributing the pills in order to reach more people who were suffering from the disease and employed between fifteen and twenty-five salesmen who rode on horseback, their saddle bags filled with pills. They covered a territory from St. Louis to Memphis and towns all along the Mississippi and Missouri Rivers, selling the pills to stores as well as to the general public. Soon the distribution area included Missouri, Arkansas, Tennessee, Kentucky, Alabama, Illinois, Indiana, Michigan, the Republic of Texas and beyond.

As the reputation grew of "Dr. Sappington's Anti-Fever Pills," as they came to be called, patients began refusing treatments from doctors who wanted to administer bleeding and purging, demanding the treatment recommended by the Missouri doctor.

Dr. Sappington wrote a book, "The Theory and Treatment of Fevers," in 1843, in order to get his message out to other physicians about the real value of quinine in the treatment of malaria. This was the first medical treatise to be published west of the Mississippi and it was sold, at Sappington's request, at a nominal price because he wanted to get it into the hands of as many people as possible.

But physicians in the medical schools continued to write in opposition to Sappington's pills for many more years, saying that his methods were too simplistic and dangerous for the common man. The debilitating and harmful methods of the time continued, probably out of stubborn jealousy that Sappington was so far ahead of his time and was enjoying such success with his simple remedy.

Dr. John Sappington made possible the travel on the Sante Fe Trail by making available his anti-fever pills at nominal prices. Because of his quinine pills and his determination to spread the knowledge about curing malaria, thousands of people lived who surely would not have otherwise.

Sappington's home and the land he developed is now a museum, near Arrow Rock, Missouri. His contribution to the health and settlement of our country is considerable and his determination for making quinine available to those who needed it is to be admired.

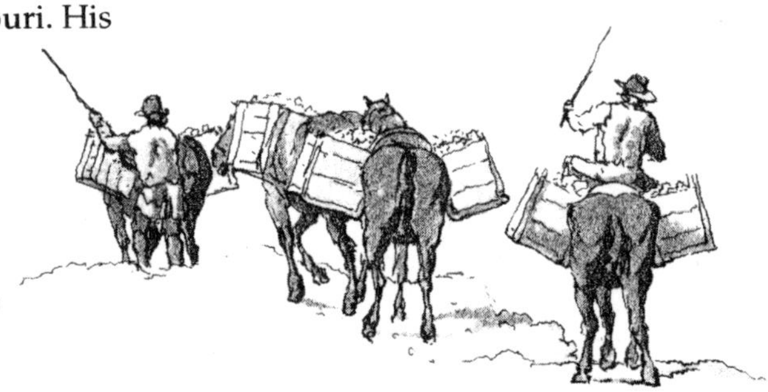

Important Advances Effecting People Who Traveled The Santa Fe Trail

1820 - Isolation of quinine from Peruvian bark by Pelletier and Caventon. Before this time, Peruvian bark was available but very unreliable as to dosage. The isolation of quinine provided accurate dosage and rapid treatment for those doctors who would accept its use.

1834 - Renucci in France found the mite that causes scabies. This disease still was claimed to be caused by "deranged humors," with bleeding and salavation (by use of mercury) used as treatment for another 20 years, however.

1836 - Quinine generally recognized as a primary treatment for malaria, although most doctors continued to practice blood-letting and purging before quinine could be administered. Many people died as a result of the stubborness of the early physicians. Patients often refused treatment that included these horrible practices.

1836 - The ascension of Queen Victoria to the throne in England. The reign of Queen Victoria is significant because England, under Victoria, soon controlled one-fourth of all the land in the world. The expansion of her Empire prompted explorers and adventurers. She funded plant-hunting expeditions into remote areas and English scientists and botanists discovered new medicines, developed mass-produced green-house glass and made important contributions to medicine. While not immediately significant to people on the Santa Fe Trail, over time the introductions of plants and medicines, as well as new sources for trade materials, did effect the lives of people who traveled along the Arkansas River and southward.

1836 - Colt revolver introduced. The use of this revolver made travel safer by offering quicker response and more defense.

1838 - *Ehrenbergs' Atlas* depicts in detail for the first time, micro-organisms and bacteria, found through the availability of newer, better microscopes.

1839 - Schonlein discovers micro-organism that causes scalp ringworm (favus). This malady was treated with all kinds of burning, and scorching compounds, accompanied by bleeding and purging, out of ignorance. Schonlein's proof of the cause was slow to change practices, but in time, radically changed treatment of favus.

1841 - Official medical treatment for malaria that the medical community recommended was changed, excluding the depletive treatments, led by Dr. Austin Flint. Dr. Flint was at least 15 years behind Dr. Sappington, who recommended immediate treatment of all ague fevers with quinine solely. However, the military recommendations for another 10 years continued to be the practice of administering purgatives and emetics.

1842 - Dr. Crawford Long in Georgia was the first to use ether as an anesthetic.

1844 - Elisha Bartlett attacks theories of Benjamin Rush (who taught excessive bleeding and purging as important to healing). The same year, Dr. Cooke, who was the Professor of Medicine at the University of Louisville Medical School, was asked to resign by his students because of his radical practices of using calomel (as much as 240 grains in 24 hours) for severe purging of patients. Patients had already been refusing treatment from this doctor and his students organized, seeking his removal from teaching at the University.

1847 - Chloroform was first used as an anesthetic.

1850 - The new Missouri Medical Association formed in St. Louis, nominating for their first president a man who had denounced the persistent uses of calomel and blood-letting. Dr. George Penn declined the nomination, refusing to be involved in the politics of the day.

1850s & '60s - Forts established along Santa Fe Trail including Forts Union, Lyon, Atkinson, Dodge, Larned and Zarah with those having physicians and hospital facilities. (Fort Bent was a civilian fort, established in 1833 and in use until 1860).

Surgeon General's Listing of Official Medical Supplies

Medical Purveyors purchased medicines and materials, based upon tables furnished by the military. Quantities of medicines, supplies and other material is given in quantities *estimated sufficient for 100 men, for one year.* The Medical Regulations list was issued in 1850 from the office of Surgeon General,Thomas Larson. Dr. Larson was from the old school supporting the depletive practices of bleeding and purging, and so, a substantial list of emetics is included. Those included alum, ipecac, tartar emetic, ammonium carbonate, zinc sulphate, senega, syrup of squill, mustard and copper sulphate.

He enforced his belief in the use of cathartics, insisting the doctors under his control use calomel, Rochele salts, Epsom salts, rhubarb, senna, Jalap, castor oil, aloes, gamboge, potassium sulphate and others. Additionally, he ordered ample supplies of lancets for bleeding and cupping glasses, scarifiers and other related instruments.

Because of Larson's beliefs in the depletive practices, and his stubborn avoidance of quinine (his recommendation for 100 men, for one year, was a total of between 2 and 12 ounces!), many field doctors carried their own supplies of quinine. Additionally, those who didn't, and followed Larson's advice, saw substantial illness and death.

Here's the official **Medical Regulations List** for 100 men, for one year:

Acacia,	4 lbs.
Acids:	
acetic	1/2 lb.
arsenic (Ars. Trioxide)	1/2 oz.
benzoic	1 oz.
Acid, citric	1 lb.
" muriatic	1/2 lb.
" nitric	1 lb.
" sulphuric	1 lb.
" aromatic	1 lb.
" tannic	2 oz.
" tartaric	2 lbs.
Etheris sulphuric loti	2 lb.
Alcohol,	cong: 5
**Aloes	4 oz.
Aluminis	1 lb.
Ammonia	1/2 lb.
*Ammoniae carbonatis	8 oz.
Ammoniaea muriatis	1/2 lb.
Anthemidis (Chamomile)	1 lb.
Antimonii et potasse, tart	3 oz.
Argenti nitratis (sil. nitrate)	2 oz.
Assafoetida	4 oz.
Camphor	2 lb.
Cantharides (blister beetle)	2 oz.
Cardamomi	8 oz.
Catechu	1/2 lb.
Cerae flavae (bees wax)	2 lb.
Cerate resin (rosin in wax)	2 lb.
Cerati simplicis (wax/lard)	8 lb.
Cerate zinc carbonate	2 lb.
**Colombo (Calumba)	5 lbs.
**Magnesium sulphate	25 lb.
*Mass of Mercury (blue mass)	8 oz.
Mellis despumati	2 lb.
Morphine sulphate	2 drm.
Myrrh	1/2 lb.
Oil anise	1 oz.
Oil clove	1 oz.
Oil cinnamon	1 oz.
Oil peppermint	1 oz.
Oil olive	8 bottle
Oil oregano	4 oz.

*Copaiba	5 lb.
Creasote	2 oz.
Cretae praep. (chalk)	1 lb.
*Copper sulphate	2 oz.
Diosmae (Buchu)	1/2 lb.
Plaster adhesive	5 yds.
" cantharides	3 lb.
" ferri	1 lb.
" hydrargyri	1/2 lb.
" resinae (rosin)	1 lb.
Ergot	2 oz.
Extract belladonna	2 oz.
*Extract colocynth comp.	8 oz
Extract licorice	6 lb.
Extract hyoscyamus	9 oz.
Ferric iodide	2 oz.
Ferric subcarbonate	4 oz.
Ferric sulphate	2 oz.
**Gambogia	1/2 oz.
Gentian	1 lb.
Glycyrrhiza (Lic. root)	1 lb.
*Hydrarg. chlor. (calomel)	1/2 oz
*Hydrarg. mitis	1 lb.
*Hydrarg. cum creta	1/2 lb.
*Hydrarg. iodidi	1 oz.
*Hydrarg. oxidi rubri	1 oz.
Iodini	2 oz.
Lini	2 oz.
Liquoris ammoniae	4 lb.
Senega	4 oz.
**Sennae	1 lb.
Serpentariae (Snakeroot)	8 oz.
Liquoris ferric iodide	1 lb.
Liquoris sodae chlor.	bot.6
Magnesium	3/4 lb.
Sodium bicarbonate	2 lb.
Sodium borate	1/2 lb.
Sodae et potassium tart.	3 lb.
Spigerliae	8oz
Spirits nitrous ether	2 lb.
Spirits of Lavender	1 lb.
Strychnine	1 drm.
*Syrup scilla	3 lb.

**Oil ricini (castor oil)	12 qt bot.
Oil turpentine	4 qt. bot.
Oil tiglii (croton)	2 drm.
Opii (Opium powder)	2 lb.
Picis abietis	1 lb.
Piperinae (pepper)	2 oz.
Plumbi acetatis (lead acetate)	1 lb.
Potassium	2 oz.
Potas. bicarbonate	1 lb.
Potas. bitartrate	1 lb.
Potas. iodide	8 oz.
Potas. nitrate (Saltpetre)	1 lb.
**Potas. sulphate	1/2 lb.
Prunus virginiana (wild cherry bark)	2 lb.
Pulveris (powdered) capsicum	1 lb.
" cinchona (peruvian bark)	1 lb.
" cubeb (green pepper)	1 lb.
* " ipecacuanha (Ipecac)	1 lb.
**Pulv. jalap	1/4 lb.
" lini	8 lb.
**Pulv. rhei (rhubarb)	1 lb.
* " sinapis nigrae (black mustard seed)	6 lb.
" ulmi (slippery elm bark)	2 lb.
Quassia (bitter ash)	1/2 lb.
Quinine sulphate	2 -12 oz.
*Rhei (rhubarb root)	1/4 lb.
Sacchari (sugar)	20 lb.
Saponis	4 lb.
Sarsaparilla	4 lb.
*Scilla	4 oz.
Tincture chloroform	1 lb.
Tincture colchium seed	1 lb.
Tincture digitalis	1/4 lb.
Tinct. ferric chloridie	1/4 lb.
Unguenti hydrargyri	1 lb.
Unguenti nitratis	1/2 lb.
Valerian	1/2 lb.
Veratriae	1/2 lb.
*Zinc sulphate	2 oz.

**Denotes emetic in the list above, while ** denotes carthartic or purgative.*

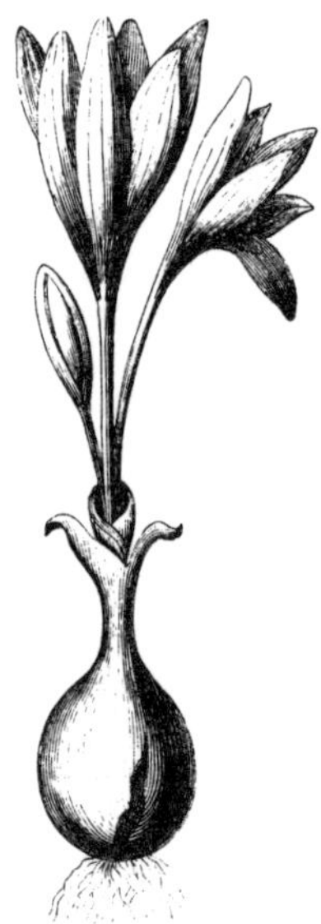

Seed and corm of Colchicum autumnale *(Crocus sativus)* was used medicinally, but only with extreme caution.

Explanation and Uses of Some of the Medicines and Herbs Listed

Acid, Acetic - Used to remove warts and corns.

Acid, Arsenic (Arsenic trioxide) - Used in chronic malaria and in cases of advanced tuberculosis.

Acid, Benzoic - can produce nausea and vomiting; somewhat sedative to the central nervous system; sometimes used in treatment of rheumatic fever, and in some cases of incontinence of urine.

Acid, Citric - It was distuinguished from tartaric and other vegetable acids in 1776 by Retzius. Scheele obtained it in crystalline form in 1784. Obtained from the not quite mature fruits of lemon, bergamot, orange, etc. Also found in cherries, raspberries, gooseberries, strawberries, etc., as well as in the roots leaves and bark of various plants. In large doses causes gastric disorder and diarrhea. Increases acidity of urine and coagulability of blood. Used as remedy for scurvy later in medicine. Used in rheumatic fever and in catarrhal jaundice.

Acid, Nitric - Lotions of nitric acid in proportion of 1/2 to 1 drachm to 1 pint of water used to arrest hemorrhage from bleeding hemorrhoids; the pure acid when touched to one or two points of a hemorrhoid sometimes produced a cure. Employed locally as a caustic for bites of rabid animals, poisonous snakes, insects and in its dilute form used for syphilitic and other sores of the mouth.

Acid, Muriatic (Hydrochloric) - The acid was first obtained in the 15th century by Basilius Valentinus and was described by him as "spirit of salt," a name that continued for some centuries. The correct composition was proved by Humphry Davy, in 1810. Found in numerous minerals and is one of the constituents of sea water. When applied in its concentrated form to the skin it causes blistering and will destroy tissue. Used to treat some forms of indigestion, and in cases of enteric fever, gastric catarrh and gastric cancer. Used in treating syphilis and in intestinal indigestion with diarrhea.

Acid, Aromatic (Sulphuric) - Sometimes called Elixir Vitrioli or Elixir of Vitriol. Has tonic and astringent properties; useful in night-sweats of phthisis, gastro-intestinal disorders. Administered diluted, followed by a mouth rinse to avoid damage to teeth.

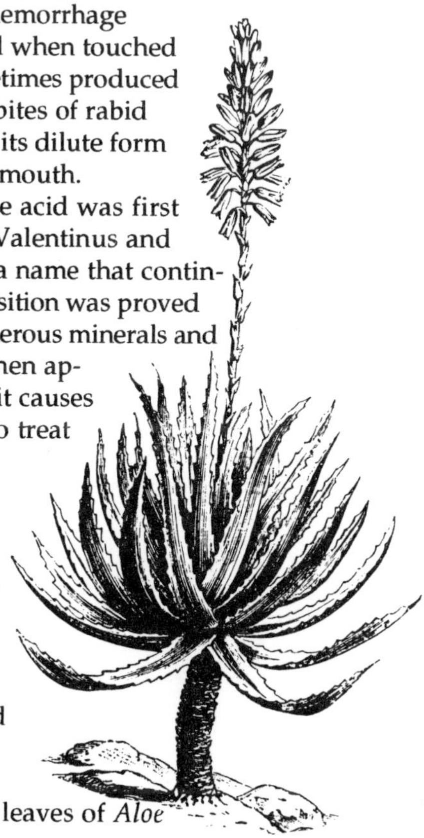

Aloes - The inspissated juice of the leaves of *Aloe*

Perryi, or *Aloe vera*, or *Aloe ferox Miller*, the later being source of Cape aloes. Native plant of eastern Africa; native aloe of southwestern U.S. also used in 19th century. Because of the bitter principle it was used as a stomachic and tonic in depraved conditions of the stomach, especially when accompanied by a sluggish liver. Aloes is a slowly acting purge and is more effective when accompanied by alkalies such as soap. Aloes increases menstrual flow; not used during pregnancy, nor in fevered states. Used in form of an enema in treatment of patients suffering from round worms and used with good result in treating chronic gonorrhea.

Aluminum/Aluminis - First isolated by Wohler in 1827; in 1854 St. Claire-Deville produced it on a commercial scale by heating sodium with the double aluminum sodium chloride. Pure aluminum has been produced only since 1890, but aluminum occurs naturally in feldspar, mica and clay, and also occurs as oxide and hydroxide and in the mineral cryolite. The entry probably refers to Aluminum sulphate, used in powder form and applied for its caustic action to cancerous growths.

Ammoniae carbonatis/Ammonium Carbonate - First prepared by Raymund Lully in the thirteenth century by the distillation of putrid urine. Subsequently obtained by the dry distillation of horn, bone, blood and other animal matters. Ammonium carbonate is similar to other preparations of ammonia in its action upon the system. If given in overdose causes gastro-enteritis, causing vomiting, purging, spinal convulsions and collapse. Moderate amounts given over a longer time produce indigestion and colicky diarrhea. Used during the course of low fevers, used alone or in combination with ammonium chloride in later states of catarrhal pneumonia, chronic bronchitis and later stages of croupous pneumonia. Alcoholic intoxication is moderated by its use; locally a solution has been used to neutralize the pain and poison of insect bites and poisonous snakes (Poisonous snakes were a worry on the Trail, but few instances of people actually being bitten by snakes are recorded. Many occurrences of animals being bitten, are recorded, however).

Anthemidis - This is the plant we know as chamomile, *Anthemis nobilis*. Other plants were substituted, including *Matricaria, Chrysanthemum parethenium*, May weed, feverfew and related plants. This plant possesses stimulant and antispasmodic properties and because of its bitter principle, acts as a simple tonic. Full doses may occasion purging, pain and vertigo. Used as a carminative in flatulent colic and in treating sick headaches and milder forms of intermittent fever. As a simple bitter the cold infusion used in anorexia during convalescence in various debilitated conditions that result in loss of appetite.

Antimonii et potasse, tart - Antimony and Potassium Tartrate. The process for the preparation was first published in 1631 by Adrian van

Mynsicht. Called Tartar emetic it was at one time used as an expectorant, diaphoretic, emetic, sedative, antiphlogistic and counterirritant. On the skin the action is that of a rubefacient and irritant. The heart rate is directly depressed by small amounts. Tartar emetic was used as a circulatory depressant in the early states of bronchitis and pneumonia, heading off colds. As an emetic it caused great prostration and muscular relaxation, but is too slow and prolonged in action to be of much use as an emetic in treating poisoning. Locally a plaster or ointment (Emplastrum antimonii) was used to treat chronically enlarged joints, applied to back of the neck for epilepsy, meningitis.

Assafoetida - Gum resins obtained from roots of *Ferula asafoetida*, a native plant of Turkey. Used as a stimulating expectorant, antispasmodic and carminative. Also sometimes used as an emmenagogue and laxative. Used in India and "Persia" as a condiment, probably because of its action to promote digestion. Given in chronic cases of constipation of the aged, often combined with other laxatives. Also used in whooping-cough, chronic bronchitis and nervous irritability of children.

Cantharides - The dried beetle, *Cantharis vesicatoria, C. vittata* and *Mylabris cichorii*, known as Cantharis or Cantharides. The insects are collected early in the morning by spreading cloth under plants, which are then shaken or beaten with poles. The insects are plunged into hot water, then spread out and dried. A better method for killing blister beetles is by means of chloroform, either or turpentine, a little being applied on cotton in a tight bottle. They were collected in July in Hungary and southern Russia, shipped in paper-lined boxes through London and New York. When swallowed they produce intense burning in the throat, stomach and bowels, with nausea and vomiting, often with bloody purging. Can cause abortion if used during pregnancy. Used in very minute doses as a stimulant for the kidneys, and as a stimulant on the skin in dry, scaly cutaneous diseases. Also employed with incontinence of urine; externally used to produce a blister when a counterirritant was desired.

Cardamomi (cardamom seed) - Used as a stomachic and carminative it relieves indigestion; also used as a spice. Usually used in a combination with other igredients, in tincture form.

Catechu - Made from the bark and sap-wood of *Acacia catechu*, a small native tree of the East Indies. Boiled for 12 hours, the wood was removed and the liquid was evaporated to form a syrup. This syrup was then spread on leaves or ashes of cow-dung, in moulds of clay and left over-night until dry, when it was broken and cut into pieces for marketing. Often combined with chalk in treatment of diarrhea and in mucous diarrhea after the patient has been thoroughly purged. Also used in treatment of uterine and vaginal leucorrhea and in chronic gonorrhea. Additional use as a dye, yielding a color known as "cutch-brown."

Cerati simplicis - Simple cerate. Made by combining white wax, 300 Gm. and benzoinated lard, 700 Gm. Used as a base for applying substances to the skin, as in salves, etc.

****Colombo** (Calumba) - From a high-climbing vine of tropical eastern Africa. In small doses used to augument secretion of liver and gastro-intestinal glands; in large doses acts as an emeto-cathartic. Produces diarrhea and sometimes vomiting and tremors. Also used as a simple bitters, during convalescence from acute infectious fevers and serous diarrhea.

***Copaiba** - Coming from any of 12 species of tropical American trees, copaiba was used as a mild stimulant, laxative and diuretic. Overdoses produced nausea, vomiting and purging. Regarded as a stimulant to mucous membranes, especially of the genito-urinary tract, used in treatment of specific urethritis and in chronic cystitis resulting from gonorrhea; used in treating hemorrhoids, applied locally to chilblains, cracked nipples, anal and other fissures. Copal varnish was used locally to abort felons, as well.

***Copper Sulphate** (Cupri sulphas) - In minute doses acts as an astringent and tonic; in full doses causes nausea and vomiting. Emetic in doses of 5 grains, but is quite poisonous in those amounts. Small doses were formerly used in treatment of chronic diarrhea and dysentery but was abandoned for internal uses due to gastro-enteritis from overdoses.

Creosote - Obtained from the distillation of wood-tar; preserved for use in tightly-stoppered dark bottles. Used to treat pulmonary tuberculosis; used as a stimulating expectorant, to relieve coughing associated with bronchitis, and in the rectum in cases of tubercular peritonitis. Used as a remedy in fermentative dyspepsia and diarrhea, and in obstinate vomiting from irritability of the stomach. Given in capsule, in wine, milk or other liquids.

Creta Preparata - Prepared chalk. A mineral mainly consisting of microscopic shells and chemically is calcium carbonate with silica, aluminum, iron, magnesium and organic matter. Used as an antacid, and for treatment of gastric problems and various forms of diarrhea. Used as an antidote to poisoning by oxalic acid; as a powder, applied in the treatment of superficial ulcers, burns, scalds and abrasions. Internally often given with mucilage or syrup.

Diosmae *(Buchu folia)* - Stimulant in certain morbid conditions of the genito-urinary tract. Was used in chronic catarrh of bladder, in chronic cystitis and as a vulnerary (in treatment of wounds) and sometimes in tincture form for flatulent dyspepsia.

Ergot - Used in medicine for two purposes: arrest of hemmorhage and contraction of dilated blood vessels.

Extract Licorice/Extract of Glycyrrhiza - Made from the root of licorice *(Glycyrrhiza glabra)*, used as a demulcent. Largely used in conjunction with infusion of flaxseed for treating coughs, sore throat, laryngitis. Also used as a flavoring to disguise the taste of other medicines. Similiar use for Licorice herb.

Extract hyoscyamus - Also called Extract of Henbane, made from the dried leaves and flowering or fruiting tops of *Hyoscyamus niger*, native of central and southern Europe. Closely allied to belladonna in action, acting more as a sedative. Combined with silver nitrate used in treating gastric ulcers and chronic gastric catarrh. Used to treat hysteria, whooping-cough and colic. When combined with purgatives is useful to prevent their griping effect. Extract in the form of a suppository frequently used to relieve pain of hemorrhoids and poultice of the leaves used to ease the pain of cancerous and other ulcers.

Gambogia (Cambogia) - Also called Gamboge or Pipe Gamboge. Seldom used except in combination with other cathartics. Used in pill, emulsion or solution made by the addition of potassium carbonate. Used in hepatic congestion, renal dropsy.

Gentian - From the dried roots of *Gentiana lutea*. Common names include bitter-root, fel-root, bitterwurzel and genciana. Classed as one of the best of the simple bitters by *The National Standard Dispensatory* as late as 1916. Excites the flow of gastric juices, promoting the appetite and aiding digestion. Used in treating loss of appetite following acute infectious diseases. Dose of the powdered drug was from 10 to 30 grains in the form of a fluidextract or tincture. Early doctors learned to use this herb from native inhabitants of North America.

Hydrargyri - Compound of Mercury. All of the compounds of mercury acted internally as an irritant poison; externally some, such as H. Ammoniatum (Ammoniated Mercury) were used for treating acute or chronic skin diseases. Hydrargyri cum creta, or Mercury with Chalk, was used for the same purpose of blue mass (Mass of Mercury), only milder in its purpose as a laxative and cholagogue. Used on children with sluggish digestion.

Iodini - Iodine. Discovered in 1811 by Courtois in the ash of seaweeds. Only known natural occurrence of iodine in free state is in Woodhall Spa Spring at Lincoln, Nebraska. Externally was sometimes used as a counterirritant over deep inflammations. Internally iodine acts as an intense gastro-intestinal irritant, producing vomiting, diarrhea. Used sometimes in tincture form in treatment of typhoid and intermittent fevers.

Myrrh - A gum-resin from any of several species of *Commiphora*. Used as a mild circulatory stimulant, and to increase the activity of the respiratory, gastric and uterine mucous membranes. Used as an expectorant in chronic bronchitis. Applied locally for spongy gums, aphtous stomatitis and indolent ulcers. Tinctures usually used for local application for ulcerative sore throat, but also given internally, as well.

Olive Oil - Also sometimes listed as sweet oil, olive oil is one of the blandest yet pleasant tasting of vegetable oils; often used as a mild laxative. Sometimes given to feeble patients to help fatten them providing their digestion was capable of dealing with oils. Used in the treatment of gall-stones, in a dose of from 1/2 to 1 pint and was claimed to soften and cause a discharge of gall-stones. Sometimes dropped into the external ear for destroying insects that found their way into the ear and also applied externally as a soothing agent for burns and skin irritation. Mixed with lime water in equal parts it forms the "Carron oil" or linimentum calcis and some cases of constipation received benefit by the injection into the bowel of olive oil at bedtime. Surgeons at one time were in the habit of dipping surgical instruments in hot olive oil before making an incision with the idea that the oil had some curative property.

Oil of Peppermint - Valued for its stimulant, carminative and anodyne properties. Used internally to treat flatulent colic, nausea and vomiting, and as an adjuvant to purgative remedies. Also useful when applied locally to treat superficial neuralgias and muscular rheumatism.

Plumbi acetatis (lead acetate) - Used as a sedative astringent; solution of lead acetate applied to mucous membranes or a broken surface of skin constringes and blanches the area and forms a white coating of lead albuminate upon it. Considered a valuable remedy in treatment of serous diarrhea and dysentery. Usually administered in pill form in combination with opium. In alcohol, in strength of 1/2 grain to the ounce of alcohol is soothing to poison ivy. Lead acetate was used in treatment of epilepsy, chorea, hysteria, aneurism and chronic bronchitis.

Potassi Nitras - Potassium Nitate, or Saltpetre, was used as far back, at least, as the eighth century. Obtained in the United States from Mammoth Cave in Kentucky and other localities. In small doses is a diuretic and diaphoretic. Larger doses produce purging and cardiac sedation. Once used in treatment of dropsy, rheumatism and fevers. For spasmodic asthma, inhalation of the fumes by way of potassium nitrate, applied to paper and rolled into cigarettes and smoked by the asthmatic, was common. Addition of tincture of benzoin or tincture of belladona, in addition to the nitre enhanced the efficiency.

Prunus virginiana - Wild cherry bark, collected from wild cherry trees throughout eastern and central North America. Used as a stomachic and bitter tonic useful in general debility. As a tonic, wild cherry was used in the form of an infusion or a fluidextract, and as a syrup. Wild cherry syrup was often used as a pleasant-tasting vehicle for other drugs.

Pulveris (powdered) capsicum - From the dried ripe fruit of *Capsicum frutescens*, or hot pepper. Applied to the skin, acts as a powerful rubefacient. Internally increases appetite and produces a sensation of heat over the entire body. Lends itself to the control of flatulence. Was generally given in combination with other remedies such as calomel and quinine to aid in their absorption and increase their efficacy. Used in treatment of intermittent fevers (not necessarily ague), as well as for simple tonsillitis pharnygitis and relaxed uvula; as gargle in treatment of scarlatina, and locally in treatment of chilblains, superficial nerualgia, rheumatism and lumbago (the latter were treated primarily with plasters of capsicum).

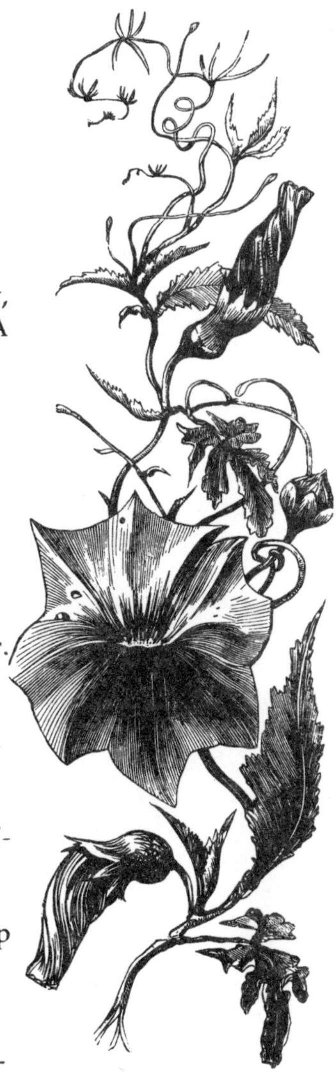

Pulveris Jalap - Jalap is the dried tuberous root of *Exogonium purga*, also listed as *Convolvulus purga*, and *Ipomea purga*, because different authors listed it differently, and because different varieties were used. A perennial climber bearing handsome rose-purple flowers similar to the cultivated morning glory. Native of the eastern slopes of the Mexican Andes, thriving at elevations of 5,000 to 8,000 feet in rainy areas. Jalap was introduced in other tropical regions, incuding India. The plants had to be at least 3 years old before harvesting was begun, and a new crop could be taken from the same plants each third year thereafter. Often dried over wood fires which gave it a slight smoky odor. Other plants with similar purgative resins that were sometimes substituted include *Ipomea orizabensis, Operculina turpenthum, Convolvulus turpenthum, Ipomea pandurata* and *Mirabilis jalapa* (the common four-o'clock). In some instances the tuber was used, and in others the seed, for the purging effect. Jalap is an active hydragogue carhartic that could cause severe griping and nausea with vomiting if given in excessive doses. Often combined with calomel as a purge; with potassium bitartrate it was used for relief of dropsy. For purging it was generally given in 5-grain doses.

Pulveris Lini (pulverized flaxseed) - Also listed as Lini semina and linseed. From the ripe seed of *Linum sativum*, an annual plant; the principle source of flax and flaxseed was Russia in the late 1800s. It was used in infusion as a demulcent for cases of acute inflammation of the gastrointestinal tract. Flaxseed acts as a soothing agent, and forms a protective coating over mucous membranes to prevent further irritation. Also used in acute bronchitis and cystitis and inflammatory conditons of the entire genito-urinary tract. Infusion was generally made by macerating 3 drachms of flaxseed and 30 grains of extract of licorice with 10 ounces of boiling water, to which was added a small quantity of lemon juice or citric acid, and sugar. Flaxseed meal was moistened with boiling water and used as a poultice.

Pulveris rhei (powdered rhubarb) - A laxative used for acid dyspepsia and some forms of diarrhea. The after-constipating effect detracts from the powder in ordinary cases of constipation. Compound powder of rhubarb was made by combining rhubarb powder, magnesium oxide and ginger, by combining the rhubarb and ginger first, mixing well in mortar, then adding the magnesia in small quantities until thoroughly mixed. German and Swiss formulas included oil of fennel in this mixture. The fresh powders had a yellowish color but gradually took on a reddish tint from the absorption of moisture and the reaction of the magnesia with the rhubarb.

Pulvenis sinapis nigrae (pulverized black mustard seed) - The dried ripe seeds of *Brassica nigra* were used like white mustard, for their laxative action. Used as a condiment, emetic and counterirritant. In small quantities it stimulates secretion of gastric juice and promotes digestion. One half to 1 tablespoonful in a pint of water, swallowed, produced vomiting and was a useful emetic in cases of poisoning. Mustard plasters were made by the addition of water or vinegar, then spread upon a piece of linen; when applied, another piece of linen was interposed between the skin and the mustard to prevent the mustard from adhering to, and burning the skin. Mustard was also often mixed with wheat flour or linseed meal. Mustard poultices were used to relieve muscular rheumatism, arthritis, neuralgia, headache. Mustard foot-bath was often used to abort forming colds, a popular remedy later in the century.

Pulveris ulmi (pulverized slippery elm bark) - The inner bark of the red elm *(Ulmus fulva)*. Slippery elm is a demulcent and used to relieve irritation of coughs, pharyngitis, laryngitis and bronchitis. In treating diarrhea, dysentery and inflammations of the urinary passages the mucilage effect of slippery elm frequently acted as a soothing, astringent agent. Poultices were also used to treat abscesses, felons and local inflammations. Internally it had a reputation as a remedy for tape worm. Slippery elm bark was popular well into the twentieth century in the form of lozenges, and are still sold in health food stores as a useful sore throat remedy.

Quasia - Listed in some sources as Bitter-wood, Bitter ash, Quassie amer, Bois amer, Quassia lignum and Lignum quassiae. Jamica quassia was derived from a small tree in the West Indies that was said to resemble an ash tree, thence the name "Bitter Ash." It is a bitter tonic, used to good benefit in dyspepsia; stimulated the appetite in anorexia following acute fevers and had similar uses as gentian and cinchona. Large doses produced vomiting.

Resin Plaster - Used to hold dressings in place and to keep edges of wounds and ends of fractured bones in place. Made of hard soap, yellow wax, dammar and rosin with a small amount of turpentine, melted together. Was spread on muslin and sold in 1 and 5 yard rolls. When exposed to great cold had a tendenancy to crack and peel off. Was prone to irritating the skin.

Saponis - Saponina, Saponins. The first use of the name saponin occurred in connection with the saponaceous constitutent of the root of Saponaria rubra, discovered by Schrader in 1808. Saponins were obtained from a variety of sources, including from Bouncing-Bet *(Saponaria officinalis), Gypsophila struthium, Arenaria rubra, Tissa rubra,* fruits of various species of *Sapindus* (called soap berries) and others. Used to treat some kinds of skin ailments and as a purgative.

Sarsaparilla - Introduced into medicine during the 16th century as a remedy for syphilis. Denounced by some doctors as useless, and by others highly highly as a specific for that disease. When given alone it exercises little influence, but in combination with mercury or ioidides it seems to increase their efficiency in-treatment of obstinate syphilis. Decoction of sarsaparilla was often recommended in chronic gout, rheumatism and sluggish skin diseases. Used as a "blood purifier"and later was a common ingredient in many patent medicines.

Scilla, Squill - Native to the Mediterannean region, the main supplies came from Malta. Because drying the plant was tedious, and qualities were often unpredictable, this was often cultivated in pharmacists' gardens. Produces a large, pear-shaped bulb, often weighing several pounds, which was sliced cross-wise and dried. The outer portions of the bulb were the most effective, with the

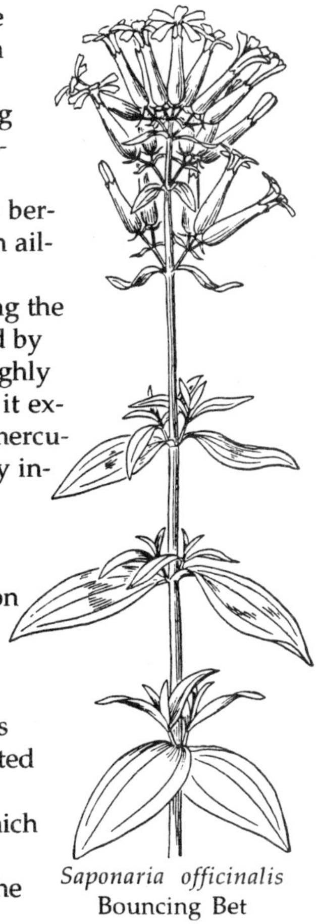

Saponaria officinalis
Bouncing Bet

new growth of the inner bulb often discarded. Used primarily for its stimulating, expectorant and diuretic properties. In the treatment of cardiac dropsy squill was frequently combined with digitalis. Administered in syrup form for bronchitis.

Senega - The dried root of *Polygala senega*, a perennial plant of eastern and central North America. Senega has a slight odor of oil of wintergreen. Other names include Seneca root, snakeroot, rattlesnake root. Used in chronic bronchitis; used for years but eventually considered useless for dropsy. Also used in spasmodic croup, after the stage of spasming subsided.

Sennae (Senna) - From the dried leaves of *Cassia acutifolia* and related plants. Sources included central Africa and the middle and upper Nile River Valley regions. Senna was considered one of the best laxatives available well into the 20th century. When used alone had a disagreeable taste and had a tendency to gripe. Usually given with fennel or coriander, or with other purgatives such as Epsom or Rochelle Salts. Simple bitters, such as gentian and colombo, increase its activity. Senna operates in about 4 hours. For constipation during pregnancy it was administered generally in the form of a compound with licorice powder. For relief of habitual constipation it was frequently combined with bitter tonics, or in infusion with fennel and Epsom Salts (the mixture later known as "Black Draught").

Spigerliae - This entry is most likely *Spigelia marilandica*, also known as Indian pink, worm-weed and pink-root. It is a native plant of the U.S., used by the medical profession since 1754 when its use was recommended by three South Carolina physicians who learned of its uses from Native Americans. Useful as an anthelmintic (meaning to destroy or expel intestinal worms), particularly if followed by a rapidly-acting purge, such as magnesium sulphate. Often given in infusion with senna, manna and fennel.

Spirits nitrous ether - Spirit of nitrous ether cools the skin, quiets nervous excitement and produces a sense of well-being. A full dose followed by a drink of hot lemonade, was a common rememdy for heading off a cold. Also used as a diuretic in cases of concentrated urine from any cause. Diuretic effect enhanced by addition of vegetable acids, citrates or tartrates.

Spirits of Lavender - Oil of lavender made by macerating lavender flowers in alcohol for 24 hours then distilling with steam. Used as a pleasant odor, and an ingredient in Florida water and lavender water; used to bathe the forehead in cases of headache and fever. Also used internally, but not to any great extent.

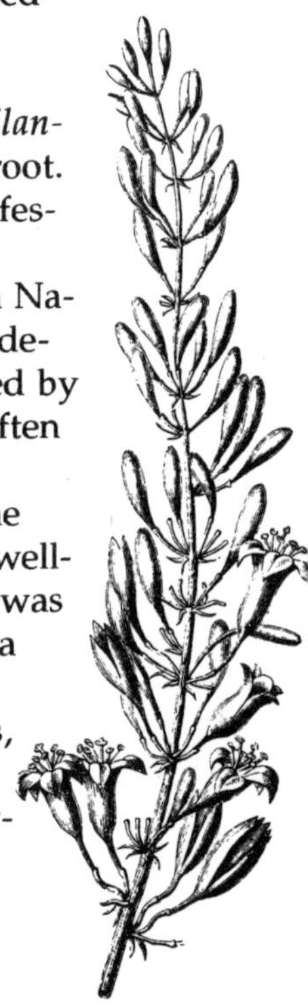

Lavandula officinalis

Tincture colchium seed - Also known as Meadow-saffron, this is from the dried corm of *Colchicum autumnale,* fall-blooming saffron crocus. Native to central and southern Europe, the seeds are the part specified in the military list, used in tincture. Both corm and seed were used medicinally. Taken in over-dose it produces violent gastro-enteritis, and possibly death. In moderately large doses caused laxity of the bowels, nausea and vomiting. The drug is one of the more dangerous poisons, because after it is taken in large doses nothing can be done to cure the patient (provided it has remained in the stomach long enough to produce its inflammatory effects). Colchicum was more prevalently used in the British Isles, common there for the treatment of gout. For the treatment of gout, tincture (sometimes called the "wine of the seed") was commonly used in a dose of from 10 to 30 minims, repeated every few hours until evidence of gastric irritation or pain in the bowels develops. The drug has been used to treat acute and chronic rheumatism, but is known, now, to have been of very little value for that. It was best used as a treatment for gout, for which it had positive effect. Most sources caution that colchicum is a powerful poison to be administered with caution.

Tincture ferric chloride - Ferric chloride was seldom used internally except in tincture form. The drug was an astringent and styptic, used to treat bleeding from tooth extraction and other minor operations, and used as a caustic and styptic for scrofulous ulcers. Given internally to arrest passive hemorrhages from the kidneys, bladder and uterus. Topical applications in diptheria and tonsillitis. Also used to some extent for chronic inflammations of mucous membreanes with diarrhea and gleet. Given in cases of follicular tonsillitis and septic infection following childbirth.

Unguenti hydrargyri (Mercurial ointment) - Made by combining mercury with benzoinated lard. Used to treat syphilis by rubbing into the skin on various parts of the body successively, as the axillae, groin, abdomen, etc. The mercury was absorbed into the body and used this way when mercury could not be administered orally, or when not easily kept on the stomach. The hands of the person applying the ointment had to be protected. This was also recommended as an application to the papules of small-pox on the face to prevent scaring. Chronic arthritis was also treated by wrapping the joint in cloths spread with the ointment. Also used as a treatment for destroying parasites infesting the region of the genitalia.

Valerian - The dried roots of the herb, *Valeriana officinalis,* native of Europe and northern Asia, cultivated in Holland, England and the United States. Valerian is used as a quieting agent in hysteria and nervousness, and for the palliation of the nervous symptoms occurring at menopause. Also shown to have benefit in treating delirium and ataxic symptoms which result from exhausting fevers. Still used as an effective home remedy as a muscle relaxer and sleep aid.

Veratriae *(Veratrum viride)* - American Hellebore or green hellebore. The dried roots of Veratrum viride was also known as itch-weed, Crow-poison and Tickle-weed. Found in the rich swamplands of eastern North America, this was a powerful sedative to the nervous, respiratory and circulatory systems. Prone to produce vomiting in over-doses, it seldom destroyed life since emesis took place so early. Abandoned as a drug due to the differing opinions as to whether it had value, but was used for a time to treat early stages of acute inflammation. The drug depresses the heat and lowers blood pressure, making it less useful in many kinds of illness.

Note: Many botanical names listed have been changed since 1850.

Itemized in the official listing of medical supplies to be procured, above, are found an abundant supply of emetics, including ipecac, alum, tartar emetic, ammonium carbonate, zinc sulphate, copper sulphate, senega, syrup of squill and mustard. Additionally, the extensive list of cathartics is apparent, including 6 mercurials including calomel, Rochelle salts, Epsom salts, potassium sulphate, rhubarb, senna, Jalap, castor oil, aloes and gamboge. The list shows how seriously behind the times the military medics were, under the leadership of Surgeon General Thomas Lawson, considering this list was issued in 1850, years after Dr. Sappington and others had demonstated the futility of purging and bloodletting.

Hospital Stores - The official listing of materials for stocking the hospital, for 100 men for one year, in 1850:

Arrow-root.................................4-10 lbs.
Barley.......................................20 lbs.
Brandy.......................................2-4 dozen bottles
Carrageen.................................1 lb.
Cinnamon..................................1/2 lb.
Cloves..4 oz.
Cocoa...10 lbs.
Ginger, ground..........................1 lb.
Molasses...................................10 gallons
Nutmegs....................................4 oz.
Tamarinds.................................6-15 lbs.
Tea...20 lbs.
Wine, bottles of........................2-4 dozen

Other hostpital supplies included 12 dozen corks, one corkscrew, 5 yards flannel, glass and tin funnels, one hatchet, ink powder, paper, inkstand, linen, lint, 1 set of medicine chests, one coffee mill, 3 mortars and pestles (including one of glass, one of iron and one of wedgewood), muslin, needles, pewter bed pan, a set of rain guages, scales and weights, sheep skins, silk, sponges, thermometers, linen thread, one 1/2 oz. box of wafers ("one to a post, two to a regiment") and sealing wax.

Major Causes of Illness

Primary diseases on the Santa Fe Trail included the ague, typhoid, smallpox, measles and cholera. The Mexican War of 1846-48 brought thousands of army troops from Fort Leavenworth and areas at the beginning of the Trail, southward to New Mexico and Mexico. Those troops brought with them diseases not found earlier in the Southwest .

In 1834, Colonel Henry Dodge led a disastrous expedition from Fort Gibson during the "sickly season," with the result of heavy casualties from malaria. The following year he commanded 3 companies of cavalry from Fort Leavenworth, during the same season (May-September) and reported a very different health record for the trip. Quinine was taken on the second trip and unofficially the army embraced the use of quinine as a preventative and treatment for malaria. Still, official medical recommendations continued to be that purgatives and emetics were of more importance, well into the 1850s. Many civilians and soldiers, alike, carried their own supplies of quinine and survived because of their forethought.

Typhoid was another matter. There was no remedy for this disease at the time. Caused by drinking contaminated water, the patient generally had to be transported in the back of a wagon until he either died or recovered. The constant movement of the wagons, with no springs or padding, over rivers, rocks, ditches and rough trails, doubtlessly hastened the deaths of many of those suffering from this disease.

Diarrhea and dysentery were constant problems due to poor food and contaminated water. Boiling water would have prevented much of the problems had the practice been known to be beneficial. Chronic problems that were a result of these illnesses haunted some people who had traveled the Trail for many years, often shortening their lives prematurely. Diarrhea came from bad food, filthy water, or a poor diet, all common complaints for the traveler.

Smallpox inoculation was discovered in 1796 by Edward Jenner. Introduced in the United States in 1800, vaccination soon became widely practiced. Still, there were outbreaks among unvaccinated groups of people, particularly among Native Americans and Mexicans who had contact with traders and soldiers. Indian tribes were disastrously affected, with heavy loss of life during the first half of the century.

Measles was also a serious threat and there were often high mortalities in the military when outbreaks occurred. The U.S. soldiers brought measles to New Mexico and Santa Fe in 1846 and epidemics caused heavy losses in many areas.

Cholera caused brief panics during the 1830s. Dr. Sappington, in Arrow Rock, Missouri, saw the first case of cholera in 1833. By 1849, between April and August, St. Louis had seen over 4,000 deaths from the disease within the city. Coal and tar were burned in quantities throughout the town in hope the smoke would drive off the pestilence, and many people fled the area entirely. Cholera ran rampant in Independence, Westport Landing and Arrow Rock, and soon traveled down the Trail. Pills made of opium, camphor, cayenne pepper and calomel were given. Rectal injections of gum arabic, laudanum and lead sugar were administered as were cantharides and mustard plasters, by doctors to people on the wagon trains, without relief. People tried anything. Cholera seemed to travel no farther south than the Arkansas River, but the towns and areas that were affected were devastated by the disease.

The Santa Fe Trail marked a profound change in American culture. With new inventions, rapdily spreading diseases, the extermination or removal of native peoples and the end of the great buffalo herds, American life would forever be altered. New medicines, many from indigenous plants as well as from plants discovered by newly-trained scientists and botanists throughout the world, new methods and new ideas opened up opportunities for expansion and population growth. Much of what was learned from the mistakes and discoveries of the first half of the 1800s would become the foundation for changes in medicine during the Civil War and beyond. Some of the same herbs and plants used on the Santa Fe Trail by the early healers, are still beneficial to us today.

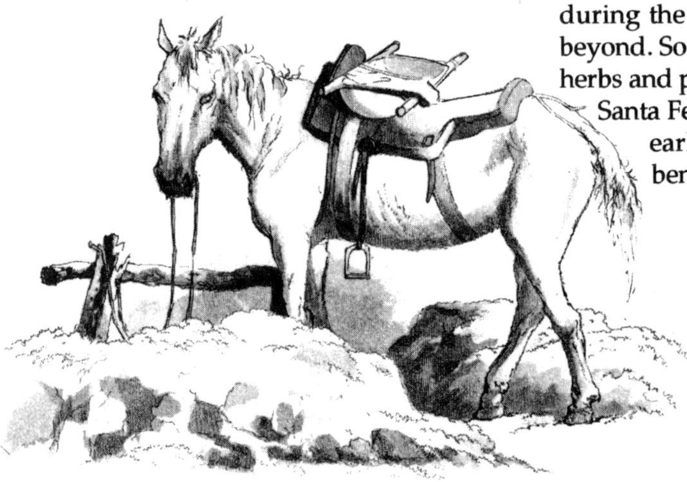

Bibliography

Collections for an Essay Towards a Materia Medica of the United States, Benjamin Smith Barton, 1798.
Commerce on the Prairies, Josiah Gregg, 1844
Down the Santa Fe Trail, The Diary of Susan Shelby Magoffin, 1846-1847
Hoblyn's Medical Dictionary, Isaac Hays, M.D., 1855
Materia Medica and Pharmacology, David Culbreth, 1927
Medicine on the Santa Fe Trail, Thomas B. Hall, M.D.
Peterson Field Guide to Medicinal Plants, Foster & Duke, 1990
Resources of the Southern Fields and Forests, a Medical Botany of the Confederate States, Francis Porcher, M.D., P.A.C.S., 1863
Squire's Companion to the British Pharmacopea, Peter Squire, 1894
The National Standard Dispensatory, 1916
The Personal Diary of Elias Slagle, 1859

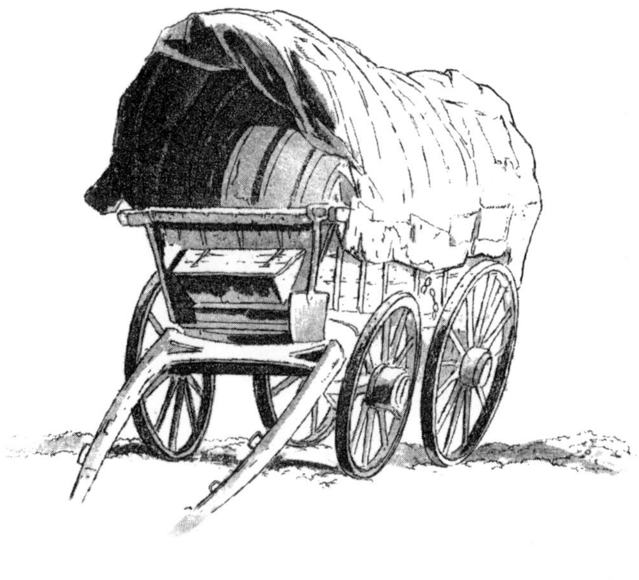

Other Books by Jim Long

Recipes & Cooking Practices of the Civil War

Herbal Cosmetics

Just for Men, Hair & Body Formulas for Men

Dream Pillows & Potions

Herbs, Just for Fun - A Beginner's Guide to Growing & Using Herbs

Tea & Cakes Under the Trellis - Making Bentwood Trellises for the Garden

Classic Blends - The Seasoning Blends of the Centuries

Successful Self-Publishing

How to Plan & Host Successful, Profitable Festivals

How to Get Free Publicity & How to Use It

How to Make Romantic Bentwood Garden Trellises, Gates, Fences & Arbors

For a complete lost of all of our books and herb products, send $2 (refundable with first order) to:
Long Creek Herbs, P.O. Box 127, Blue Eye, Missouri 65611
www.Longcreekherbs.com

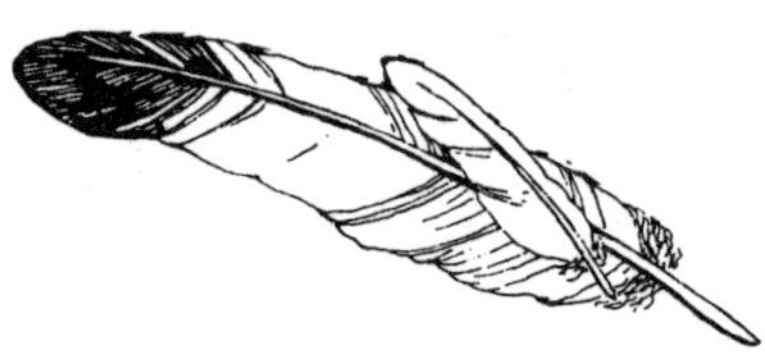